Fast Pegan Diet Cookbook for Beginners

Super Tasty, Affordable and Quick Recipes for Busy People

Emy Fit

Table of Contents

Greek Potato Salad

Preparation time: 10minutes

Cooking time: 20minutes

Servings: 3

Ingredients:

- 6 potatoes, scrubbed or peeled and chopped

- Salt

- 1/4 cup olive oil

- 2 tablespoons apple cider vinegar

- 2 tablespoons freshly squeezed lemon juice

- 1 teaspoon dried herbs

- 1/2 cucumber, chopped

- 1/4 red onion, diced

- 1/4 cup chopped pitted black olives

- Freshly ground black pepper

Directions:

1. Set the potatoes in a pot, add a pinch of salt, and pour in enough water to cover. Boil the water. Cook the potatoes for 15 to 20 minutes, until soft. Drain and set aside to cool. (Alternatively, put the potatoes in a large microwave-safe dish with a bit of water. Cover and heat on high power for 10 minutes.)

2. In a large bowl, whisk together the olive oil, vinegar, lemon juice, and dried herbs. Toss the cucumber, red onion, and olives with the dressing.
3. Add the cooked, cooled potatoes, and toss to combine. Taste and season with salt and pepper as needed.

Nutrition: Calories: 110 Fats: 17.1g, Carbs: 19.6g Fiber: 7.5g Sugar: 17.1g Proteins: 7.6g Sodium: 121mg

Pesto and White Bean Pasta Salad

Preparation time: 15minutes

Cooking time: 10minutes

Servings: 4

Ingredients:

- 1.1/2 cups canned cannellini beans

- 1/2 cup Spinach Pesto

- 1 cup chopped tomato or red bell pepper

- 1/4 red onion, finely diced

- 1/2 cup chopped pitted black olives

Directions:

1. In a large bowl, combine the pasta, beans, and pesto. Toss to combine.

2. Add the tomato, red onion, and olives, tossing thoroughly.

Nutrition:

Calories: 110

Fats: 17.1g,

Carbs: 19.6g

Fiber: 7.5g

Sugar: 17.1g

Proteins: 7.6g

Sodium: 121mg

Mediterranean Orzo and Chickpea Salad

Preparation time: 15minutes

Cooking time: 8minutes

Servings: 4

Ingredients:

- 1/4 cup olive oil

- 2 tablespoons freshly squeezed lemon juice

- Pinch salt

- 1.1/2 cups canned chickpeas, drained and rinsed

- 2 cups orzo or other small pasta shape, cooked according to the package directions, drained, and rinsed
with cold water to cool

- 2 cups raw spinach, finely chopped

- 1 cup chopped cucumber

1/4 red onion, finely diced

•

Directions:

1. In a large bowl, whisk together the olive oil, lemon juice, and salt. Add the chickpeas and cooked orzo, and toss to coat.

2. Stir in the spinach, cucumber, and red onion.

Nutrition:

Calories: 110

Fats: 17.1g,

Carbs: 19.6g

Fiber: 7.5g

Sugar: 17.1g

Proteins: 7.6g

Sodium: 121mg

Vegetable Stir-Fry

Preparation Time: 10minutes

Cooking time: 15minutes

Servings: 4

Ingredients:

- Zucchini (.50)

- Red Bell Pepper (.50)

- Broccoli (.50)

- Red Cabbage (1 C.)

- Brown Rice (.50 C.)

- Tamari Sauce (2 T.)

- Red Chili Pepper (1)

- Fresh Parsley (.25 t.)

- Garlic (4)

- Olive Oil (2 T.)

- Optional: Sesame Seeds

Directions:

1. To begin, you will want to cook your brown rice according to the directions that are placed on the package. Once this step is done, place the brown rice in a bowl and put it to the side.

2. Next, you will want to take a frying pan and place some water in the bottom. Bring the pan over medium heat and then add in your chopped vegetables. Once in place, cook the vegetables for five minutes or until they are tender.

3. When the vegetables are cooked through, you will then want to add in the parsley, cayenne powder, and the garlic. You will want to cook this mixture for a minute or so. Be sure you stir the ingredients so that nothing sticks to the bottom of your pan.

4. Now, add in the rice and tamari to your pan. You will cook this mixture for a few more minutes or until everything is warmed through.

5. For extra flavor, try adding sesame seeds before you enjoy your lunch! If you have any left-overs, you can

keep this stir-fry in a sealed container for about five days in your fridge.

Nutrition:

Calories: 280

Protein: 10g

Fat: 12g

Carbs: 38g

Fibers: 6g

Broccoli Over Orzo

Preparation Time: 10minutes

Cooking time: 25minutes

Servings: 3

Ingredients:

- Olive Oil (3 t.)

- Smashed Garlic Cloves (4)

- Broccoli Florets (2 C.)

- Orzo Pasta (4.50 Oz.)

- Salt (.25 t.)

- Pepper (.25 t.)

Directions:

1. Start off by preparing your broccoli. You can do this by trimming the stems off and slicing the broccoli into small, bite-size pieces. If you want, go ahead and season with salt.

2. Next, you will want to steam your broccoli over a little bit of water until it is cooked through. Once the broccoli is cooked, chop it up into even smaller pieces.

3. When the broccoli is done, cook your pasta according to the directions provided on the box. Once this is done, drain the water and then place the pasta back into the pot.

4. With the pasta and broccoli done, place it back into the pot with the garlic. Stir everything together well and cook until the garlic turns a nice golden color. Be sure to stir everything to combine your meal well. Serve warm and enjoy a simple dinner!

Nutrition:

Calories: 230

Protein: 10g

Fat: 5g

Carbs: 39g

Fibers: 5g

Miso Spaghetti Squash

Preparation Time: 5minutes

Cooking time: 50minutes

Servings: 4

Ingredients:
- 1 (3-pound) spaghetti squash

- 1 tablespoon hot water

- 1 tablespoon unseasoned rice vinegar

- 1 tablespoon white miso

Directions:

1. Preheat the oven.

2. Peel the squash, cut-side down, on the prepared baking sheet. Bake for 35 to 40 minutes, until tender.

3. Cool until the squash is easy to handle. With a fork, scrape out the flesh, which will be stringy, like spaghetti. Transfer to a large bowl.

4. In a small bowl, combine the hot water, vinegar, and miso with a whisk or fork. Pour over the squash. Gently toss with tongs to coat the squash.

5. Divide the squash evenly among 4 single-serving containers. Let cool before sealing the lids.

6. Storage: Place in the refrigerator for up to 1 week or freeze for up to 4 months. To thaw, refrigerate overnight. Reheat in a microwave for 2 to 3 minutes.

Nutrition:

Calories: 120

Protein: 10g

Fat: 16g

Carbs: 79g

Fibers: 5g

Garlic and Herb Oodles

Preparation Time: 5minutes

Cooking time: 2minutes

Servings: 3

Ingredients:

- 1 teaspoon extra-virgin olive oil or 2 tablespoons vegetable broth

- 1 teaspoon minced garlic (about 1 clove)

- 4 medium zucchinis, spiraled

- 1/2 teaspoon dried basil

- 1/2 teaspoon dried oregano

- 1/41/4 to 1/2 teaspoon red pepper flakes, to taste

- 1/4 teaspoon salt (optional)

- 1/4 teaspoon freshly ground black pepper

Directions:

1. Heat the olive oil. Add the garlic, zucchini, basil, oregano, red pepper flakes, salt (if using), and black pepper. Sauté for 1 to 2 minutes, until barely tender.

2. Divide the oodles evenly among 4 storage containers. Let cool before sealing the lids.

Nutrition:

Calories: 120

Protein: 10g

Fat: 44g
Carbs: 32g

Fibers: 5g

Baked Brussels Sprouts

Preparation Time: 10minutes

Cooking time: 40minutes

Servings: 4

Ingredients:

- 1 pound Brussels sprouts

- 2 teaspoons extra-virgin olive or canola oil

- 4 teaspoons minced garlic (about 4 cloves)

- 1 teaspoon dried oregano

- 1/2 teaspoon dried rosemary

- 1/2 teaspoon salt

- 1/4 teaspoon freshly ground black pepper

- 1 tablespoon balsamic vinegar

Directions:

1. . Preheat the oven to 400°F.

2. Trim and halve the Brussels sprouts. Transfer to a large bowl. Toss with the olive oil, garlic, oregano, rosemary, salt, and pepper to coat well.

3. Transfer to the prepared baking sheet. Bake for 35 to 40 minutes, shaking the pan occasionally to help with even browning, until crisp on the outside and tender on the inside.

4. Remove from the oven and transfer to a large bowl. Stir in the balsamic vinegar, coating well.

5. Divide the Brussels sprouts evenly among 4 single-serving containers. Let cool before sealing the lids.

Nutrition: Calories: 128 Protein: 10g Fat: 50g Carbs: 23g Fibers: 5g

Roasted Herb Carrots

Preparation Time: 10minutes

Cooking time: 25minutes

Servings: 4

Ingredients:

- 21/2 pounds carrots, quartered

- 2 tablespoons olive oil or avocado oil

- 1/4 cup Clean Ranch Seasoning, or store-bought light or low-sodium ranch dressing
- mix Salt

- Freshly ground black pepper

Directions:

1. Preheat the oven to 425°F. Line a baking sheet with aluminum foil.

2. On the prepared baking sheet, toss the carrots with the olive oil. Sprinkle with the ranch seasoning and season with salt and pepper. Shake the pan so the carrots are in a single layer.

3. Roast for 25 minutes, or until browned and bubbly.

4. 4.

5. Let cool and portion the carrots into 4 single-serving 24-ounce meal prep containers. Refrigerate for up to 5 days.

Nutrition:

Calories: 191;

Fat: 7g;

Protein: 2g;

Total carbs: 31g;

Net carbs: 22g;

Fiber: 7g;

Sugar: 14g;

Sodium: 234mg

Gluten-Free, Vegan Banana Pancakes

Preparation Time: 10 minutes

Cooking time: 5 minutes

Servings: 2-3

Ingredients:

- 1 cup generally useful, gluten-free flour

- 1/2 tsp. preparing powder

- 1/2 tsp. cinnamon dash ocean salt

- 1 tsp. apple juice vinegar

- 2/3 cup almond milk

- 1 ready banana

- 1 teaspoon vanilla

- 1 tbsp. + 2 tsp. dissolved coconut oil, isolated

Directions:

1. Mix the flour, preparing powder, cinnamon, and ocean salt together.

2. Mix the vinegar to the almond milk and whisk together till foam. Include the almond/vinegar blend to a blender, alongside the banana, vanilla, and 1 tbsp. coconut oil. Mix till smooth.
3. Mix the fluid blend into the flour blend till consolidated.

4. Warm 2 tsp. coconut oil in a nonstick skillet. Include the hitter, storing 1/4 cup at once. Give the hotcakes a chance to cook till air pockets structure on the top; at that point, flip and keep cooking till flapjacks are cooked through. Rehash with all outstanding hitter.

5. Serve flapjacks with new berries.

Nutrition:

Calories: 122;

Fat: 19g;
Protein: 13g;

Carbohydrates: 54g;

Fiber: 25g;

Sugar: 10g;

Sodium: 124mg

Apple Cinnamon Oatmeal

Preparation Time: 5 minutes

Cooking time: 0 minutes

Servings: 2

Ingredients:

- 1 cup gluten-free moved oats

- 1 cup of water

- 3/4 cup almond milk

- 3/4 cup diced apples

- 1/2 teaspoon cinnamon or pumpkin pie zest

- 2 tbsp. maple syrup

- 1/4 cup slashed crude pecan pieces

Directions:

1. Add the oats, water, almond milk, apples, cinnamon, and syrup in a medium pot or pan. Heat to the point of boiling and lower to a stew. Cook until oats have assimilated. The fluid and apples are delicate (around 10-15 minutes).

2. Divide oats into two dishes and top with crude pecan pieces. Appreciate.

Nutrition:

Calories: 122;

Fat: 2g;

Protein: 43g;

Carbohydrates: 64g;

Fiber: 95g;

Sugar: 17g;

Sodium: 224mg

Pumpkin Spice Overnight Oats

Preparation Time: 5 minutes

Cooking time: 0minutes

Servings: 1

Ingredients:

- 1/2 t. vanilla

- 3/4 t. pumpkin spice

- 3 to 4 drops liquid stevia

- 1 tbsp. chia seed

- 2 tbsp. canned pumpkin puree

-
  1/2 c. hemp hearts
- 1/3 c. of the following:

- Brewed coffee

- Almond milk unsweetened vanilla silk

Directions:

1. In a bowl with a lid, add all the ingredients, mixing until well-combined.

2. Cover and refrigerate overnight or 8 hours.

3. Remove from the fridge and add additional milk until the oats reach your desired consistency.

4. Divide into 2 bowls and enjoy.

Nutrition:

Calories: 132

Proteins: 6.5 g

Carbohydrates: 4.9 g

Fats: 1 g

Crab with Spicy Seeds

Preparation time: 5 minutes

Cooking time: 20 minutes

Servings: 6

Ingredients:

- 1 cup sunflower seeds

- Seeds for cupping cups

- 1/2 cup chia seeds

- 1/2 cup sesame (I used a mixture of black and white sesame)

- 1 copper (starch) seeds

- 1 cup of water 1 1/2

- Selected 1 tablespoon dried herbs

- 1 tea spoon of peppers standard, (optional)

Directions:

1. Preheat the oven to 170° C.

2. Mix all ingredients and let the seeds float in water for 10-15 minutes.

3. Mix well, then divide the mixture into two baking trays and lightly grease. The ideal thickness is about 3-4 mm. They are very thin, the cakes are very weak, very thick, and more like granular cakes.
4. Bake every time (partially change the dishes) or until golden and crispy. If you do not feel an explosion after an hour, return to the oven for another 5-10 minutes.

5. Remove from the oven, cool and press into rough places. Storage in stored containers.

Nutrition:

Calories: 5

Fat: 19 g

Protein: 18g

Sodium: 101mg

Fiber: 6 g

Carbohydrates: 187g
Sugar: 1.4 g

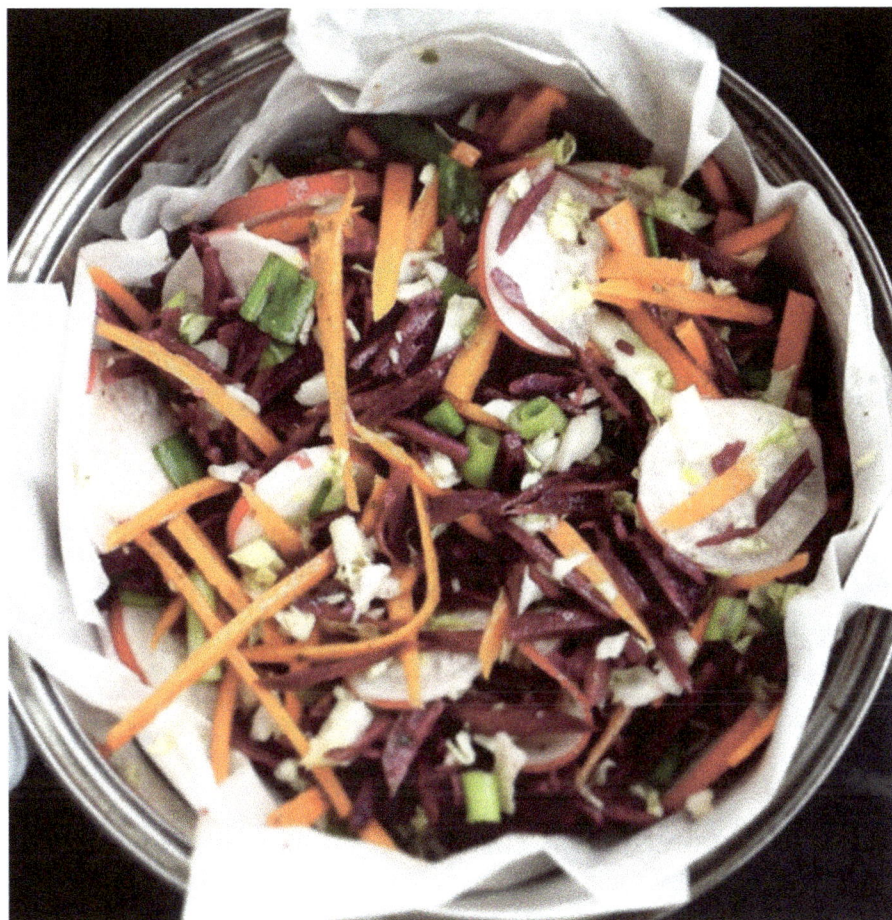

Sweet Potato Slaw in Wonton Cups

Preparation time: 15 minutes

Cooking time: 20minutes

Servings: 5

Ingredients:

- 1 cup water

- 2 cups sliced green cabbage (roughly 1 small head)

- 1 cup shredded sweet potato

- 1/2 sweet onion, sliced

- 2 tablespoons lite soy sauce

- 1 tablespoon hoisin sauce

- 11/2 tablespoons freshly squeezed lime juice

- 11/2 teaspoons sesame oil

- Zest of 1 lime

- 1/2 teaspoon ground ginger, plus more to taste

- 3 scallions, green and light green parts, sliced

Directions:

1. Preheat the oven to 350°F. Lightly coat a muffin tin with the nonstick spray.

2. Place one wonton wrapper in each well of the prepared tin, pressing down to create a cup shape. Bake for 5 to 6 minutes, or until the cups are crispy and lightly browned. Set aside to cool.

Nutrition:

Calories: 5

Fat: 19 g

Protein: 17g

Sodium: 11mg

Fiber: 8 g

Carbohydrates: 54g

Sugar: 1.4 g

Mediterranean Cod Stew

Preparation Time: 10 minutes

Cooking time: 20minutes

Servings: 6

Ingredients:

- 2 tablespoons olive oil

- 2 cups chopped onion (about 1 medium onion)

- 2 garlic cloves, minced (about 1 teaspoon)

- 3/4 teaspoon smoked paprika

- 1 can diced tomatoes,

-
  1 jar roasted red peppers
- 1 cup sliced olives, green or black

- 3/4 cup dry red wine

- 1/4 teaspoon black pepper

- 1/4 teaspoon kosher

- 1.1/2 pounds cod fillets,

- 3 cups sliced mushrooms

Directions:

1. Heat the pot and heat the oil. Attach the onion and cook.

2. Attach the garlic and smoked paprika and cook.

3. Mix in the tomatoes with their juices, roasted peppers, olives, wine, pepper, and salt, and turn the heat up to medium-high. Bring to a boil. Add the cod and mushrooms, and reduce the heat to medium.

4. Cook in a low heat and, stir for a few times, until the cod is cooked through and flakes easily, and serve.

Nutrition:

Calories: 223

Total Fat: 4g

Saturated Fat: 9g

Cholesterol: 7

Sodium: 45mg

Total Carbohydrates: 8g

Fiber: 3g; Protein: 6g

Steamed Mussels in White Wine Sauce

Preparation Time: 5 minutes

Cooking time: 10minutes

Servings: 4

Ingredients:

- 2 pounds small mussels

- 1 tablespoon extra-virgin olive oil

- 1 cup sliced red onion

- 3 garlic cloves, sliced

- 1 cup dry white wine

- 2 (1/4-inch-thick) lemon slices

- 1/4 teaspoon freshly ground black pepper

- 1/4 teaspoon kosher or sea salt

- Fresh lemon wedges, for serving (optional)

Directions:

1. In a large colander in the sink, run cold water over the mussels (but don't let the mussels sit in standing water). All the shells should be closed tight; discard any shells that are a little bit open or any shells that are cracked. Leave the mussels in the colander until you're ready to use them.

2. Heat the oil in a skillet. Attach the onion and cook,

3. Add the mussels and cover. Cook in a low heat.

4. All the shells should now be wide open. Using a slotted spoon, discard any mussels that are still closed. Spoon the opened mussels into a shallow serving bowl, and pour the broth over the top.

Serve with additional fresh lemon slices, if desired.

Nutrition:

Calories: 123

Total Fat: 7g

Saturated Fat: 9g

Cholesterol: 15

Sodium: 45mg

Total Carbohydrates: 8g

Fiber: 3g; Protein: 6g

Orange and Garlic Shrimp

Preparation Time: 10 minutes

Cooking time: 20minutes

Servings: 5

Ingredients:

- 1 large orange

- 3 tablespoons extra-virgin olive oil, divided

- 1 tablespoon chopped fresh rosemary

- 1 tablespoon chopped fresh thyme (about 6 sprigs) or 1 teaspoon dried thyme

- 3 garlic cloves, minced (about 11/2 teaspoons)

- 1/4 teaspoon freshly ground black pepper

- 1/4 teaspoon kosher or sea salt

  11/2 pounds fresh raw shrimp, (or frozen and thawed raw shrimp) shells and tails removed

•

Directions:

1. Zest the entire orange using a Micro plane or citrus grater.

2. Using a zip-top bag, merge the orange zest and 2 tablespoons of oil with the rosemary, thyme, garlic, pepper, and salt. Attach the shrimp, seal the bag, and gently massage the shrimp.
3. . Heat a grill, grill pan, or a large skillet over medium heat. Brush on or swirl in the remaining 1 tablespoon of oil. Add half the shrimp, and cook for 4 to 6 minutes, or until the shrimp turn pink and white, flipping halfway through if on the grill or stirring every minute if in a pan.

4. While the shrimp cook, peel the orange and cut the flesh into bite-size pieces. Serve immediately or refrigerate and serve cold.

Nutrition:

Calories: 223

Total Fat: 7g

Saturated Fat: 10g

Cholesterol: 45

Sodium: =15mg

Total Carbohydrates: 8g

Fiber: 3g; Protein: 6g

Roasted Shrimp-Gnocchi Bake

Preparation Time: 10 minutesCooking time: 20minutes

Servings: 6

Ingredients:

- 1 cup tomato

- 2 tablespoons extra-virgin olive oil

- 2 garlic cloves, minced

- 1/2 teaspoon black pepper

- 1/4 teaspoon crushed red pepper

- 1 jar red peppers

- 1-pound fresh raw shrimp

- 1-pound frozen gnocchi

- 1/2 cup cubed feta cheese

- 1/3 cup fresh torn basil leaves

Directions:

1. Preheat the oven to 425°F.

2. In a baking dish, mix the tomatoes, oil, garlic, black pepper, and crushed red pepper. Roast in the oven for 10 minutes.

3. Stir in the roasted peppers and shrimp. Roast for 10 more minutes, until the shrimp turn pink and white.

4. While the shrimp cooks, cook the gnocchi on the stove top according to the package directions. Drain in a colander and keep warm.

5. Remove the dish from the oven. Mix in the cooked gnocchi, feta, and basil, and serve.

Nutrition:

Calories: 223

Total Fat: 7g

Saturated Fat: 16g

Cholesterol: 25

Sodium: =10mg

Total Carbohydrates: 8g

Fiber: 3g; Protein: 6g

Spicy Shrimp Puttanesca

Preparation Time: 5 minutes

Cooking time: 15minutes

Servings: 4

Ingredients:

- 2 tablespoons extra-virgin olive oil

- 3 anchovy fillets, drained and chopped (half a 2-ounce tin), or 11/2 teaspoons anchovy paste

- 3 garlic cloves, minced (about 11/2 teaspoons)

- 1/2 teaspoon crushed red pepper

- 1 (14.5-ounce) can low-sodium or no-salt-added diced tomatoes, untrained

- 1 (2.25-ounce) can sliced black olives, drained (about 1/2 cup)

- 2 tablespoons capers
1 tablespoon chopped fresh oregano or 1 teaspoon dried oregano

-

- 1-pound fresh raw shrimp (or frozen and thawed shrimp), shells and tails removed

Directions:

1. In a large skillet over medium heat, heat the oil. Mix in the anchovies, garlic, and crushed red pepper. Cook for 3 minutes, stirring frequently and mashing up the anchovies with a wooden spoon, until they have melted into the oil.

2. Stir in the tomatoes with their juices, olives, capers, and oregano. Turn up the heat to medium-high, and bring to a simmer.

3. When the sauce is lightly bubbling, stir in the shrimp. Reduce the heat, and cook the shrimp and serve.

Nutrition:

Calories: 423

Total Fat: 7g

Saturated Fat: 16g

Cholesterol: 25

Sodium: =55mg

Total Carbohydrates: 34g

Fiber: 3g;

Protein: 6g

Burrito & Cauliflower Rice Bowl

Preparation Time: 15 minutes

Cooking Time: 10 minutes

Servings: 4

Ingredients:

- 1 cup cooked tofu cubes

- 12 oz. frozen cauliflower rice

- 4 teaspoons olive oil

- 1 teaspoon unsalted taco seasoning

- 1 cup red cabbage, sliced thinly

- 1/2 cup salsa

- 1/4 cup fresh cilantro, chopped

- 1 cup avocado, diced

Directions:

1. Prepare cauliflower rice according to directions in the package.

2. Toss cauliflower rice in olive oil and taco seasoning.
3. Divide among 4 food containers with lid.
4. Top with tofu, cabbage, salsa and cilantro.
5. Seal the container and chill in the refrigerator until ready to serve.
6. Before serving, add avocado slices.

Nutrition:

Calories 298

Total Fat 20 g

Saturated Fat 3 g
Cholesterol 0 mg

Sodium 680 mg

Total Carbohydrate 15 g

Dietary Fiber 6 g

Total Sugars 5 g

Protein 15 g

Super food Buddha Bowl

Preparation Time: 10 minutes

Cooking Time: 10 minutes

Servings: 4

Ingredients:

- 8 oz. microwavable quinoa

- 2 tablespoons lemon juice

- 1/2 cup hummus

- Water

- 5 oz. baby kale

- 8 oz. cooked baby beets, sliced

- 1 cup frozen shelled edam me (thawed)

- 1/4 cup sunflower seeds, toasted

- 1 avocado, sliced

- 1 cup pecans

- 2 tablespoons flaxseeds

Directions:

1. Cook quinoa according to directions in the packaging.

2. Set aside and let cool.

3. In a bowl, mix the lemon juice and hummus.

4. Add water to achieve desired consistency.

5. Divide mixture into 4 condiment containers.

6. Cover containers with lids and put in the refrigerator.

7. Divide the baby kale into 4 food containers with lids.

8. Top with quinoa, beets, Edam me and sunflower seeds.

9. Place in the refrigerator until it's ready.

Nutrition:

Calories 381

Total Fat 19 g

Saturated Fat 2 g

Cholesterol 0 mg

Sodium 188 mg

Total Carbohydrate 43 g

Dietary Fiber 13 g
Total Sugars 8 g

Protein 16 g

Potassium 1,066 mg

Grilled Summer Veggies

Preparation Time: 15 minutes

Cooking Time: 6 minutes

Servings: 6

Ingredients:

- 2 teaspoons cider vinegar

- 1 tablespoon olive oil

- 1/4 teaspoon fresh thyme, chopped

- 1 teaspoon fresh parsley, chopped

- 1/4 teaspoon fresh rosemary, chopped

- Salt and pepper to taste

- 1 onion, sliced into wedges

- 2 red bell peppers, sliced

- 3 tomatoes, sliced in half

- 6 large mushrooms, stems removed

- 1 eggplant, sliced crosswise

- 3 tablespoons olive oil

- 1 tablespoon cider vinegar

Directions:

1. Merge the vinegar, oil, thyme, parsley, rosemary, salt and pepper to make the dressing.

2. In a bowl, mix the onion, red bell pepper, tomatoes, mushrooms and eggplant.

3. Toss in remaining olive oil and cider vinegar.

4. Grill over medium heat for 3 minutes.

5. Turn the vegetables and grill for another 3 minutes.

6. Arrange grilled vegetables in a food container.

7. Drizzle with the herbed mixture when ready to serve.

Nutrition:

Calories 127

Total Fat 9 g

Saturated Fat 1 g

Cholesterol 0 mg

Sodium 55 mg

Total Carbohydrate 11 g

Dietary Fiber 5 g

Total Sugars 5 g

Protein 3 g

Potassium 464 mg

"Cheesy" Spinach Rolls

Preparation Time: 20 minutes

Cooking Time: 15 minutes

Servings: 6

Ingredients:

- 18 spinach leaves

- 18 vegan spring roll wrappers

- 6 slices cheese, cut into 18 smaller strips

Water

- 1 cup vegetable oil

- 6 cups cauliflower rice

- 3 cups tomato, cubed

- 3 cups cucumber, cubed

- 1 tablespoon olive oil

- 1 teaspoon balsamic vinegar

Directions:

1. Add one spinach leaf over each wrapper.

2. Add a small strip of vegan cheese on top of each spinach leaf.

3. Roll the wrapper and seal the edges with water.

4. In a pan over medium high heat, add the vegetable oil.

5. Cook the rolls until golden brown.

6. Drain in paper towels.

7. Divide cauliflower rice into 6 food containers.

8. Add 3 cheesy spinach rolls in each food container.

9. Toss cucumber and tomato in olive oil and vinegar.

Nutrition: Calories 746 Total Fat 38.5g Saturated Fat 10.1g Cholesterol 33mg Sodium 557mg
Total Carbohydrate 86.2g Dietary Fiber 3.8g Total Sugars 2.6g Protein 18g Potassium 364mg

Pesto Pasta

Preparation Time: 10 minutes

Cooking Time: 8 minutes

Servings: 2
Ingredients:

- 1 cup fresh basil leaves

- 4 cloves garlic

- 2 tablespoons walnut

- 2 tablespoons olive oil

- 1 tablespoon vegan Parmesan cheese

- 2 cups cooked penne pasta

- 2 tablespoons black olives, sliced

Directions:

1. Put the basil leaves, garlic, walnut, olive oil and Parmesan cheese in a food processor.

2. Pulse until smooth.

3. Divide pasta into 2 food containers.

4. Spread the basil sauce on top.

5. Top with black olives.

6. Store until ready to serve.

Nutrition:

Calories 374

Total Fat 21.1g

Saturated Fat 2.6g

Cholesterol 47mg

Sodium 92mg

Total Carbohydrate 38.6g

Dietary Fiber 1.1g

Total Sugars 0.2g

Protein 10g

Potassium 215mg

Tofu Sharma Rice

Preparation Time: 15 minutes

Cooking Time: 15 minutes

Servings: 4

Ingredients:

- 4 cups cooked brown rice

- 4 cups cooked tofu, sliced into small cubes

- 4 cups cucumber, cubed

- 4 cups tomatoes, cubed

- 4 cups white onion, cubed

- 2 cups cabbage, shredded

- 1/2 cup vegan mayo

- 1/8 cup garlic, minced

- Garlic salt to taste
- Hot sauce

Directions:

1. Add brown rice into 4 food containers.

2. Arrange tofu, cucumber, tomatoes, white onion and cabbage on top.

3. In a bowl, mix the mayo, garlic, and garlic salt.

4. Drizzle top with garlic sauce and hot sauce before serving.

Nutrition: Calories 667 Total Fat 12.6g Saturated Fat 2.2g Cholesterol 0mg Sodium 95mg

Total Carbohydrate 116.5g Dietary Fiber 9.9g
Total Sugars 9.4g Protein 26.1g Potassium 1138mg

Risotto with Tomato & Herbs

Preparation Time: 10 minutes

Cooking Time: 20 minutes

Servings: 32

Ingredients:

- 2 oz. Arborio rice

- 1 teaspoon dried garlic, minced

- 3 tablespoons dried onion, minced

- 1 tablespoon dried Italian seasoning, crushed

- 3/4 cup snipped dried tomatoes

Directions:

1. Make the dry risotto mix by combining all the ingredients except broth in a large bowl.

2. Divide the mixture into eight resalable plastic bags. Seal the bag.

3. Store at room temperature for up to 3 months.

4. When ready to serve, pour the broth in a pot.

5. Add the contents of 1 plastic bag of dry risotto mix.

6. Bring to a boil and then reduce heat.

7. Bring with vegetables.

Nutrition:

Calories 80

Total Fat 0 g

Saturated Fat 0 g

Cholesterol 0 mg
Sodium 276 mg

Total Carbohydrate 17 g

Dietary Fiber 2 g

Total Sugars 0 g

Protein 3 g

Potassium 320 mg

Vegan Tacos

Preparation Time: 20 minutes

Cooking Time: 10 minutes

Servings: 4

Ingredients:

- 1/2 teaspoon onion powder

- 1/2 teaspoon garlic powder

- 1 teaspoon chili powder

- 2 tablespoons tamari

- 16 oz. tofu, drained and crumbled

- 1 tablespoon olive oil

- 1 ripe avocado

- 1 tablespoon vegan mayonnaise

- 1 teaspoon lime juice

- Salt to taste

- 8 corn tortillas, warmed

- 1/2 cup fresh salsa

- 2 cups iceberg lettuce, shredded

- Pickled radishes

Directions:

1. Merge all the ingredients in a bowl.

2. Marinate the tofu in the mixture for 10 minutes.

3. Pour the oil in a pan over medium heat.

4. Cook the tofu mixture for 10 minutes.

5. In another bowl, mash the avocado and mix with mayo, lime juice and salt.

6. Stuff each corn tortilla with tofu mixture, mashed avocado, salsa and lettuce.

7. Serve with pickled radishes.

Nutrition:

Calories 360

Total Fat 21 g

Saturated Fat 3 g

Cholesterol 0 mg

Sodium 610 mg

Total Carbohydrate 33 g
Dietary Fiber 8 g

Total Sugars 4 g

Protein 17 g

Potassium 553 mg

Spinach with Walnuts & Avocado

Preparation Time: 5 minutes

Cooking Time: 0 minute

Servings: 1

Ingredients:

- 3 cups baby spinach

- 1/2 cup strawberries, sliced

- 1 tablespoon white onion, chopped

- 2 tablespoons vinaigrette

- 1/4 medium avocado, diced

- 2 tablespoons walnut, toasted

Directions:

1. Put the spinach, strawberries and onion in a glass jar with lid.

2. Drizzle dressing on top.

3. Top with avocado and walnuts.

4. Shut down the lid and refrigerate until ready to serve.

Nutrition: Calories 296 Total Fat 18 g Saturated Fat 2 g Cholesterol 0 mg Sodium 195 mg

Total Carbohydrate 27 g Dietary Fiber 10 g Total Sugars 11 g Protein 8 g Potassium 103 mg

Roasted Veggies in Lemon Sauce

Preparation Time: 15 minutes

Cooking Time: 20 minutes

Servings: 5

Ingredients:

- 2 cloves garlic, sliced

- 1 .1/2 cups broccoli florets

- 1 .1/2 cups cauliflower florets

-
  1 tablespoon olive oil
- Salt to taste

- 1 teaspoon dried oregano, crushed

- 3/4 cup zucchini, diced

- 3/4 cup red bell pepper, diced

- 2 teaspoons lemon zest

Directions:

1. Preheat your oven to 425 degrees F.

2. Merge the garlic, broccoli and cauliflower.

3. Put in the oil and season with salt and oregano.

4. Roast in the oven for 10 minutes.

5. Attach the zucchini and bell pepper to the pan.

6. Stir well.

7. Roast for another 10 minutes.

8. Sprinkle lemon zest on top before serving.

9. Fill to a food container and reheat before serving.

Nutrition: Calories 52 Total Fat 3 g Saturated Fat 0 g Cholesterol 0 mg Sodium 134 mg Total Carbohydrate 5 g Dietary Fiber 2 g Total Sugars 2 g Protein 2 g

Tender Lamb Chops

Preparation Time: 10 Minutes

Cooking Time: 3 Hours

Servings: 4

Ingredients:

- 8 lamb chops

- ½ teaspoon dried thyme

- 1 onion, sliced

- 1 teaspoon dried oregano

- 2 garlic cloves, minced

- 4 baby carrots

- Pepper and salt

- 2 potatoes, cubed

- 8 small tomatoes, halved

Directions:

1. Add the onion, carrots, tomatoes and potatoes into a pot.

2. Combine together thyme, oregano, pepper, and salt. Rub over lamb chops.

   2. Place lamb chops in the pot and top with garlic.
   3. Pour ¼ cup water around the lamb chops.
   4. Cover and cook on low flame for around 3 hours.
   5. Uncover the pot and roast at high flame for 10 minutes.
   6. Serve and enjoy.

Nutrition:

Calories 210

Fat 4.1 g

Carbohydrates 7.3 g

Protein 20.4 g

Beef Stroganoff

Preparation Time: 10 Minutes

Cooking Time: 4 Hours

Servings: 2

Ingredients:

- 1/2 lb. beef stew meat

- 10 oz mushroom soup, homemade

- 1 medium onion, chopped

- 1/2 cup sour cream

    oz mushrooms, sliced
- Pepper and salt

Directions:

1. Add all fixings excluding sour cream into a pot and mix well.

2. Cover and cook on low flame for 4 hours.
3. Add sour cream and stir well.
4. Serve and enjoy.

Nutrition:

Calories 470

Fat 25 g

Carbohydrates 8.6 g

Protein 49 g

Lamb & Couscous Salad

Preparation Time: 7 Minutes

Cooking Time: 25 Minutes

Servings: 2

Ingredients:

- 1/2 Cup Water

- 1/2 Tablespoon Garlic, Minced

- 1 1/4 lb. Lamb Loin Chops, Trimmed

- 1/4 Cup Couscous, Whole Wheat

- Pinch Sea Salt

- 1/2 Tablespoon Parsley, Fresh & Chopped Fine

- 1 Tomato, Chopped
-
  1 Teaspoon Olive Oil
- 1 Small Cucumber, Chopped

- 1 1/2 Tablespoons Lemon Juice, Fresh

- 1/4 Cup Feta, Crumbled

  1 Tablespoon Dill, Fresh & Chopped Fine

•

Directions:

1. Get out a saucepan and bring the water to a boil.

2. Get out a bowl and mix your garlic, salt and parsley. Press this mixture into the side of each lamb chop, and then heat your oil using medium-high heat in a skillet.

3. Add the lamb, cooking for six minutes per side. Place it to the side, and cover to help keep the lamb chops warm.

4. Stir the couscous into the water once it's started to boil, returning it to a boil before reducing it to low so that it simmers. Cover, and then cook for about two minutes more. Take away from heat, then allow it to stand uncovered for five minutes. Fluff using a fork, and then add in your tomatoes, lemon juice, feta and dill. Stir well. Serve on the side of your lamb chops.

Nutrition:

Calories: 232,

Fat: 7.9g,

Protein: 5.6g,

Carbohydrates: 31.2g

Smoky Pork & Cabbage

Preparation Time: 10 Minutes

Cooking Time: 3 Hours

Servings: 6

Ingredients:

3lb pork

1/2 cabbage head, chopped

1 cup water

1/3 cup liquid smoke

1 tablespoon kosher salt

Directions:

1. Rub the pork with kosher salt and place into a pot.

2. Pour liquid smoke over the pork. Add water.
3. Cover then cook on low flame for 2 hours.
4. Remove pork from the pot and add cabbage in the bottom.
5. Place pork on top of the cabbage.
6. Cover again and cook for 1 hour more.
7. Slice the pork and serve.

Nutrition:

Calories 484

Fat 21.5 g

Carbohydrates 4 g

Protein 36 g

Banana and Almond Butter Oats

Preparation Time: 10 minutes

Cooking time: 5 minutes

Servings: 2

Ingredients:

- 1 cup gluten-free moved oats

- 1 cup almond milk

- 1 cup of water

- 1 teaspoon cinnamon

- 2 tablespoons almond spread

- 1 banana, cut

Directions:

1. Mix the water and almond milk to a bubble in a little pot. Add the oats and diminish to a stew.

2. Cook until oats have consumed all fluid. Blend in cinnamon. Top with almond spread and banana and serve.

Nutrition:

Calories: 112;

Fat: 10g;

Protein: 9g;

Carbohydrates: 54g;

Fiber: 15g;

Sugar: 5g;

Sodium: 180mg

Greek Flatbreads

Preparation time: 15minutes

Cooking time: 10minutes

Servings: 4

Ingredients:

- 4 *Pita Bread* rounds or store-bought pita rounds

- 2 cups baby spinach leaves

- 1 cup sliced grape tomatoes

- 1/2 cup pitted, halved Klamath olives

- 1/2 cup thinly sliced red onion

- 1/3 cup thinly sliced fresh basil

- 1/4 cup sliced Greek pepperoncini (optional)

- 3 tablespoons extra-virgin olive oil (optional)

Directions:

1. Preheat the oven to 350°F.

2. Set the pita rounds on the oven rack and bake for 5 to 10 minutes until lightly browned and crisp.

3. Place a pita on each plate. Spread the hummus evenly over each. Evenly distribute the spinach, tomatoes, olives, onion, basil, and pepperoncini (if using) on top. Drizzle with olive oil (if using), then cut into quarters and serve immediately.

Nutrition:

Calories: 437

Total fat: 7g

Protein: 82g

Sodium: 346

Fat: 19g

Mediterranean Macro Plate

Preparation time: 10minutes

Cooking time: 10minutes

Servings: 4

Ingredients:

- 6 cups cauliflower florets

- 8 ounces firm or extra-firm tofu

- Olive oil cooking spray

- 1 tablespoon herbs de Provence

- Sea salt

- 1 recipe Full Madams

- *1* recipe Happy Hummus

- 6 cups sliced cucumber

Directions:

1. Spout an inch of water into a large pot and insert a steamer rack. Bring the water to a boil, add the cauliflower, cover, and cook over medium heat until tender, about 10 minutes.

2. While the cauliflower is cooking, cut the tofu into 1-inch cubes. Heat a large skillet over medium-high heat. Spray with cooking spray and lay the tofu in a single layer in the skillet. Sprinkle evenly with the herbs de Provence and salt. Cook for 4 minutes, or until the undersides are golden brown. Spray with cooking spray, flip, and cook for an additional 3 to 4 minutes until golden brown on the other side. Remove from the heat.

3. Divide the full me dames and hummus among 6 plates. Add a scoop of tofu and cauliflower to each plate and divide the cucumber for dipping into the hummus. Serve immediately.

Nutrition:

Calories: 537

Total fat: 7g

Protein: 82g

Sodium: 446

Fat: 19g

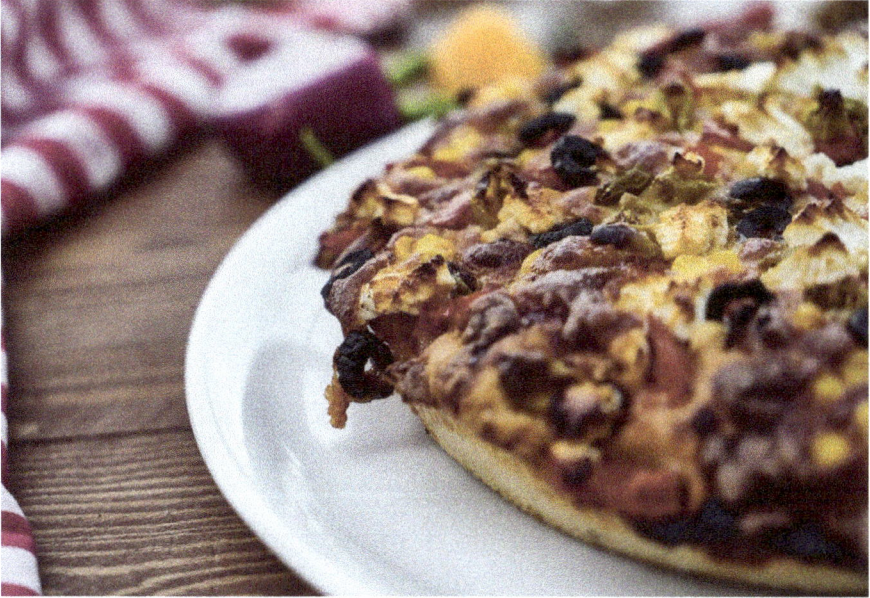

The Athena Pizza

Preparation time: 10minutes
Cooking time: 15minutes

Servings: 3

Ingredients:

- 4 *Pita Bread* rounds or store-bought pita bread

- 6 cups lightly packed stemmed and thinly sliced kale

- 2 tablespoons freshly squeezed lemon juice

- 1 tablespoon extra-virgin olive oil

- 4 garlic cloves, finely minced or pressed

- 1/4 teaspoon sea salt

- 1 recipe Macadamia-Rosemary Cheese

- 1 cup halved grape or cherry tomatoes

  1/2 cup pitted, chopped Klamath olives

•

Directions:

1. Preheat the oven to 400°F.

2. Arrange the pita bread rounds in a single layer on two large rimmed baking sheets. Bake for 5 to 10 minutes until golden brown and crisp. Remove and set aside.

3. In a large bowl, mix the kale, lemon juice, and olive oil. Using your hands, work the lemon and oil into the kale, squeezing firmly, so that the kale becomes soft and tenderized, as well as a darker shade of green. Stir in the garlic and salt.

4. . Assemble the pizzas by spreading each pita with a generous coating of macadamia cheese and topping evenly with the kale salad, tomatoes, and olives.

Nutrition:

Calories: 537

Total fat: 7g

Protein: 82g

Sodium: 446

Fat: 19g

Bream

Preparation time: 10minutes

Cooking time: 60minutes

Servings: 4

Ingredients:

- Olive oil cooking spray

- 2 medium zucchinis, cut into 1/2inch-thick rounds

- 2 gold potatoes, thinly sliced

- 4 tomatoes, sliced

- 1.3/4 cups tomato sauce

- 10 garlic cloves cut into large chunks

- 1.1/2 tablespoons olive oil

- 4 teaspoons dried basil

- 2 teaspoons dried oregano
- Teaspoon sea salt

Directions:

1. In a large bowl, combine the zucchini, potatoes, tomatoes, tomato sauce, garlic, olive oil, basil, oregano, and salt and stir well. Pour the vegetable into the dish.

2. Bake for 30 minutes, stir well, and bake for another 30 minutes, or until the potatoes are tender. Stir again and serve.

Nutrition:

Calories: 337

Total fat: 8

Protein: 82g

Sodium: 346

Fat: 19g

Green-Glory Soup (Pot)

Preparation time: 10 minutes

Cooking time: 15 minutes

Servings: 4

Ingredients:

- 1 head cauliflower (florets)

- 1 onion (diced)

- 2 cloves garlic (minced)

- 1 cup spinach (fresh or frozen)

- 1 bay leaf (crumbled)

- 1 cup coconut milk

- 4 cups vegetable stock

- Salt and pepper to taste

- Herbs for garnish (optional)

- 1/2 cup coconut oil

Directions:

1. In a pressure pot on "sauté" mode, sauté onions and garlic until onions are browned. Once cooked, add the cauliflower and bay leaf and cook for about 5 minutes, stirring occasionally.

2. Add the spinach and continue cooking and stirring for 5 minutes.

3. Pour in the vegetable stock and set the timer for 10 minutes on high pressure to let the mix come to a boil; then allow quick pressure release and add the coconut milk.

4. Season with garnishes of choice as well as salt and pepper. Turn off the pot and mix the soup until it becomes thick and creamy with a hand blender.

Nutrition:

Calories: 114

Total fat: 9g

Saturated fat: 5g

Sodium: 128mg

Carbs: 19g

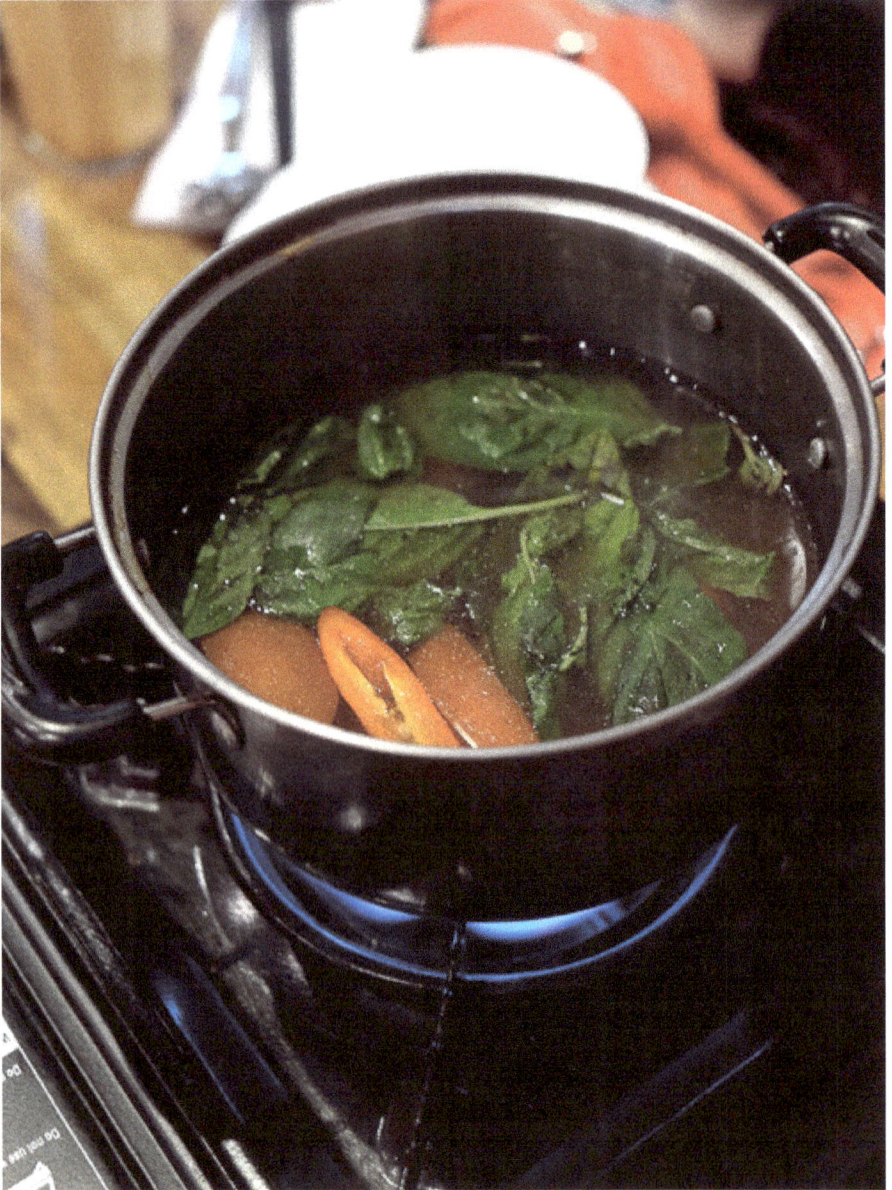

Fiber: 8g

Protein: 6g

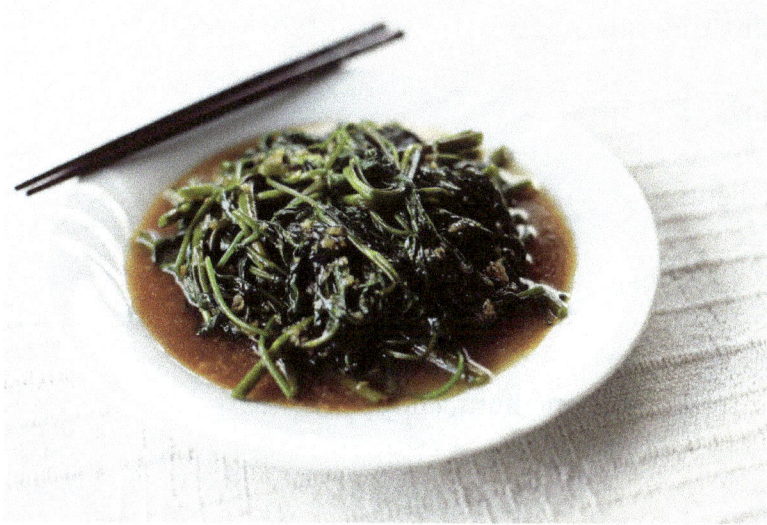

Veggie Soup (Pot)

Preparation time: 5 minutes

Cooking time: 10 minutes

Servings: 4

Ingredients:

- 2 tbsp. olive oil

- 1 onion (medium, chopped)

- 3 tbsp. parsley (fresh, minced)

- 1 clove of garlic (minced)

- 3 (14.5 oz.) cans vegetable broth

- 4 cups tomatoes (chopped)

- 1 cup celery (chopped)

- 1 cup carrots (sliced)

- 1 zucchini (halved and sliced)

- 2 tsp. basil (dried, crushed)

- 1/2 tsp. salt

- 1/2 tsp. Italian seasoning

- 1 tsp. red pepper flakes (crushed)

- 5 cups kale leaves (chopped)

Directions:

1. Heat pot on "sauté" mode until it says "hot"; then adds the oil.

2. Attach the onion, and cook until it is tender. Add the parsley and garlic, stirring constantly for 30 seconds; then add the vegetable broth.

3. Stir in the celery, tomato, zucchini, carrots, Italian seasoning, and red pepper to the pot and turn off the heat. Close the lid.

4. Turn the steam option to "sealing," selecting high pressure for 6 minutes. When done, turn the cooker

off again, choosing the quick pressure release option; then select "sauté."

5. Add kale, stirring for 3 minutes or so until the soup comes to a boil. Turn the cooker off and serve.

Nutrition: Calories: 134 Total fat: 9g Saturated fat: 5g Sodium: 138mg Carbs: 26g Fiber: 8g Protein: 6g

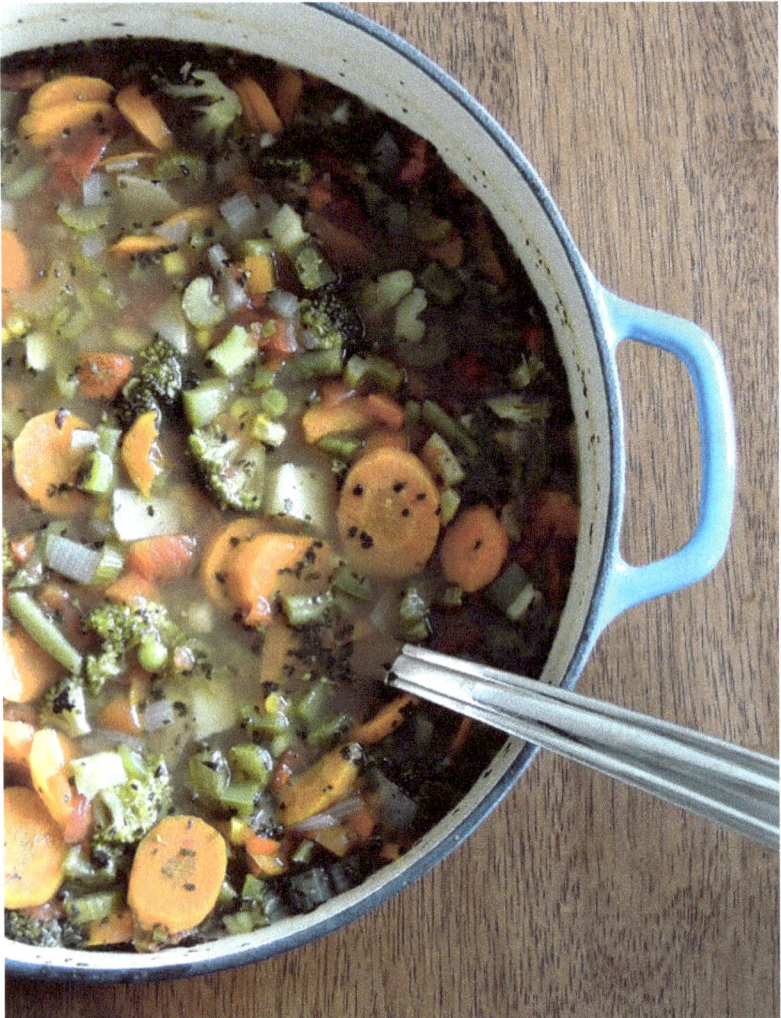

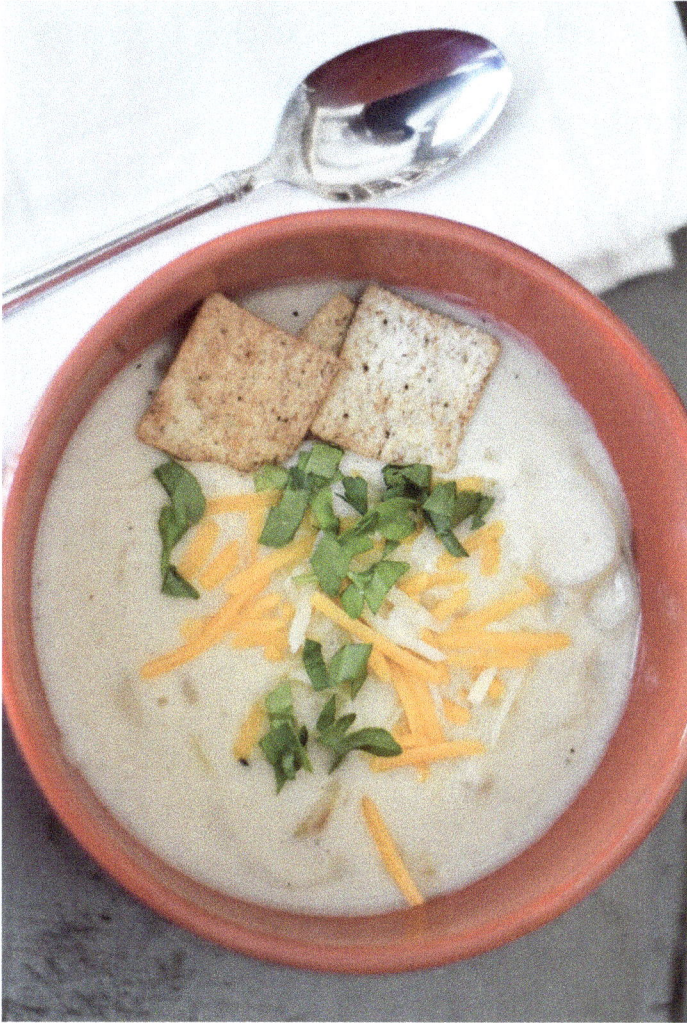

Creamy Italian Herb Soup

Preparation time: 10 minutes

Cooking time: 30 minutes
Servings: 4

Ingredients:

- 2 cans full fat coconut milk

- 1/2 cup coconut cream

- 1/4 cup fresh parsley

- 1 cup broccoli florets

- 1 cup veggie broth

- 1 tbsp. olive oil

- 1 tsp. nutritional yeast

- 1 finely chopped onion

  2 cloves minced garlic

- •

- • 1 cup fresh Italian herbs (basil, oregano, rosemary, thyme, and sage)

- • Salt and black pepper to taste

Directions:

1. Caramelize onion and garlic in a large cooking pan over medium heat.

2. Add Italian herbs, stir, and adding coconut milk while stirring.

3. Add remaining ingredients with salt and pepper to taste and cook for 30 minutes.

4. You can blend it after cooking or eat it when it's the right temperature.

5. If you want to store and freeze, you have to blend it.

6. Either transfers it directly to a heat safe blender, or let it cool, then blends until smooth.

Nutrition: Calories: 124 Total fat: 9g Saturated fat: 5g Sodium: 118mg Carbs: 16g Fiber: 8g Protein: 6g

Cauliflower Soup (Pot)

Preparation time: 10 minutes

Cooking time: 30 minutes

Servings: 4

Ingredients:

- 3 cups vegetable stock

- 2 tsp. thyme powder

- 1/2 tsp. match green tea powder

- 1 head cauliflower (about 2.5 cups, florets)

- 1 tbsp. olive oil

- 5 garlic cloves (minced)

- Salt and pepper to taste

Directions:

1. In an pressure pot, add the vegetable stock, thyme, and match powder on medium heat. Bring to a boil.

2. Add the cauliflower and set timer for 10 minutes on high pressure, allowing for quick pressure release when finished.

3. In a saucepan, add garlic and olive oil until tender and you can smell it; then add it to the pot along with salt and cook for 1 to 2 minutes.

4. Turn off the heat and. blend the soup and creamy with a blender.

Nutrition:

Calories: 114

Total fat: 9g

Saturated fat: 5g

Sodium: 128mg

Carbs: 18g

Fiber: 8g

Protein: 6g

Lasagna Soup

Preparation time: 5 minutes

Cooking time: 30 minutes

Servings: 5

Ingredients:

- Vegetable broth – 2 cups

- Portobello mushrooms, gills removed and finely diced – 8 ounces

- Onion powder – 1 teaspoon

- Crushed tomatoes – 28 ounces

- Diced tomatoes – 28 ounces

- Olive oil – 2 tablespoons

- Garlic, minced – 4 cloves

- Basil, fresh, chopped - .33 cup

- Nutritional yeast – 2 tablespoons

- Sea salt – 1 teaspoon

- Lentil Lasagna noodles (Explore Cuisine) – 8 ounces

- Vegan mozzarella shreds - .66 cup

- Thyme, dried – 1 teaspoon

Directions:

1. Pour the olive oil and allow it to heat over medium-high. Add in the diced mushrooms and cook while stirring regularly for eight minutes. Pour the diced tomatoes, garlic, and basil into the pot and continue to cook for four minutes.

2. Into the soup pot, add the crushed tomatoes, onion powder, thyme, nutritional yeast, and vegetable broth. Bring this mixture to a boil. Crack the lasagna noodles into small pieces and add them into the pot. Reduce the heat, fit on a lid, and allow the soup to simmer on low for twenty minutes.

3. Serve the soup topped with the vegan mozzarella shreds.

Nutrition:

Calories: 134

Total fat: 9g

Saturated fat: 5g

Sodium: 118mg

Carbs: 19g

Fiber: 9g

Protein: 6g

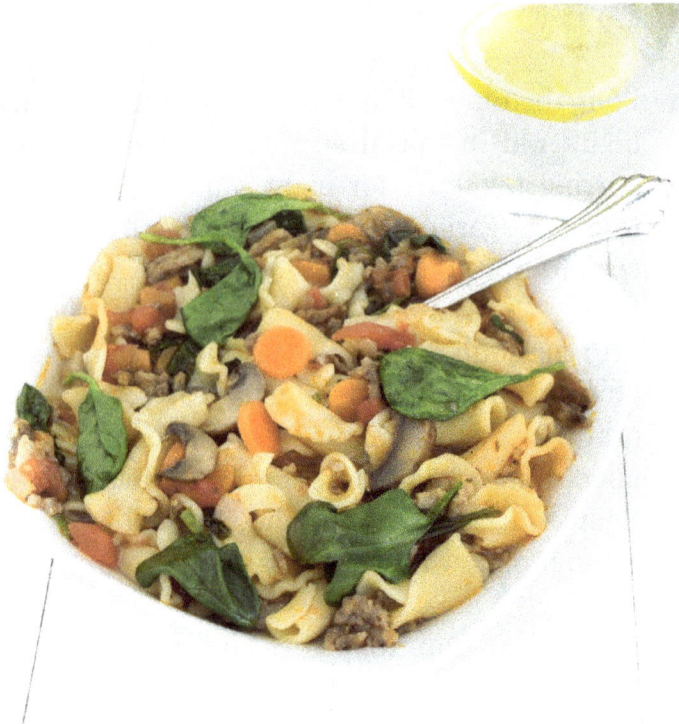

Tabbouleh Salad

Preparation time: 5minutes

Cooking time: 12minutes

Servings: 4

Ingredients:

- 1/4 cup olive oil

- 2 tablespoons freshly squeezed lemon juice

- 2 garlic cloves, minced

- Pinch salt

- Pinch freshly ground black pepper

- 2 tomatoes, diced

- 1/2 cup chopped fresh parsley

- Cup dry bulgur wheat, cooked according to the package directions

Directions:

1. Merge together the olive oil, lemon juice, garlic, salt, and pepper. Gently stir in the tomatoes and parsley.

2. Attach the bulgur and toss to combine everything thoroughly. Taste and season with salt and pepper as needed.

Nutrition:

Calories: 110

Fats: 12.1g,

Carbs: 15.6g

Fiber: 7.5g

Sugar: 17.1g

Proteins: 7.6g

Sodium: 121mg

Caesar Salad

Preparation time: 10minutes

Cooking time: 0minutes

Servings: 4

Ingredients:

- 2 cups chopped romaine lettuce
- 2 **tablespoons** Caesar Dressing

- 1 serving *Herbed Croutons* or store-bought croutons

- Vegan cheese, grated (optional)

- Make it a meal

- 1/2 cup cooked pasta

- 1/2 cup canned chickpeas

- 2 additional tablespoons *Caesar Dressing*

Directions:

1. To make the Caesar salad

2. Merge together the lettuce, dressing, croutons, and cheese (if using).

3. To make it a meal

4. Add the pasta, chickpeas, and additional dressing. Toss to coat.

Nutrition: Calories: 120 Fats: 13.1g, Carbs: 12.6g Fiber: 7.5g Sugar: 17.1g Proteins: 7.6g Sodium: 121mg

www.ingramcontent.com/pod-product-compliance
Lightning Source LLC
Chambersburg PA
CBHW050746030426
42336CB00012B/1677